Praise for *Healing*

"A tonic for the afflicted with cancer or otherwise. For patients, caregivers, and the public."

—Barry Boyd, MD
Greenwich Hospital, Yale New Haven Health System

"Jerry Rhine has written a compelling narrative of transformation and resilience in the face of life threatening illness. This book is a reflection on what actions and thoughts made a difference in Jerry's own emotional and physical survival. A valuable and personal read for those of us facing similar challenges in life."

—Steven F. Horowitz, MD, FACC
Cardiology Chief at Beth Israel
Cardiology Chief at Stamford Hospital

"A wonderful example of how dedicated practice of imagery and spirituality facilitates recovery from devastating physical and mental illness. Jerry Rhine's remarkable recovery from stroke and cancer reminds us all of the powerful role mind-set and imagery plays in healing from diseases deemed unreachable by psychological intervention"

—Jeffrey Deitz, MD
psychiatrist & psychoanalyst
author of *Intensive Therapy*

"We can all learn from those who have preceded us on this difficult journey called life. Jerry Rhine's visualizations and experience can be your guide and coach when you encounter life's difficulties and help you to survive and thrive."

—Dr. Bernie Siegel, MD
Yale University
author of *The Art of Healing and A Book of Miracles*
Saul Presser University of Pennsylvania

"I am a practicing gastroenterologist having studied at Harvard. I recently came across an interesting book by Jerry Rhine (Healing); this is an important book. After 30 years of practice, I am always amazed at the power of the mind in ameliorating symptoms of inflammatory bowel disease and irritable bowel syndrome. I have seen patients with similar disease have far different outcomes. We used to call it nervous colitis, because those who had poor outcomes appeared to be mentally challenged in handling their disease and in some circles it was thought that they actually brought the disease on themselves.

It was actually the power of the brain in conjunction with the person's ability to utilize it and produce the needed neurotransmitters and endorphins to mollify the disease in those who had good outcomes. I feel it does have a place in dealing with patient care."

—Sharon Lattig
Professor of English, University of Connecticut

"Wonderful and insightful book. I highly recommend it for people looking for an alternative approach. I give it 5 Stars."

—Dr. Alan Rosenthal
University of Pennsylvania

"Insightful, hopeful and helpful book by a man who has lived it."

—Alfred Wolfson, MD
Yale New Haven Hospital

"What is so powerful in this work is how the author walks us gently through those aspects of our humanity so crucial to healing when life seems to exists as if only being held by a thread—courage, compassion, giving, forgiveness, hope. Through the technique of visualization he leads us to the integration of our experiences for transformation. The author writes of his journey of healing, saying I have been there and survived, and you will too. . . . A must read."

—Dr. Karen Shields
Catholic spiritual director, Fordham University

"I recommend Jerry Rhine's book to all who are traveling challenging paths. Jerry has the creativity and skill to make the journey less difficult and, perhaps even, a ladder to greater connection to that inner light within each of us. He is a knowledgeable and compassionate companion."

—Rabbi M. J. Newman
Jewish and Palliative Care Chaplain, Greenwich Hospital,
Yale New Haven Health Services member

"*Healing* is a simple yet profound book that will help you to find the solutions to not only healing yourself from illness but creating a life of well being, peace and happiness. Beautiful full color pictures and illustrations make this book a joy to read. This book is powerful because Jerry Rhine has lived the advice that he is sharing with you. . . . This book is a must read for everyone. Don't wait till you are dealing with a disease in your life. If you want happiness and healing this is the book for you."

—Lionel R. Ketchian

"This science based book can help adolescents who are challenged by education, socialization, separation, and pressure to succeed. The result of these stressful dramatic changes in their lives often leads to poor moods. The images reflecting positive emotional states can help reverse their anxiety and depression."

—Sharon Lattig
Professor of English, University of Connecticut

"Jerry Rhine's book *Healing* is must for any person faced with the challenge of heart disease or cancer, it is an inspirational read and helps patients keep positive and inspired during their difficult journeys."

—Joseph Feuerstein, MD
Director of Integrative Medicine, Stamford Hospital,
Assistant Clinical Professor of Medicine, Columbia University

"*Healing* is an excellent book written by a cancer and heart disease survivor. Through techniques such as meditation and visualization . . . patients can contribute to their own healing. These methodologies are presently underutilized but can add hope and years to patients who otherwise can fall into despair and depression."

—Dr. Saul Presser
University of Pennsylvania

"The simplicity and honesty within this book make it stand out as an invaluable and inspiring guide for people confronting any illness. This book is ultimately a personal story of Jerry Rhine's own healing from cancer and heart disease. That is what makes this book more meaningful and powerful. The love and determination he demonstrated in his healing process models to all of us how we too can become better people and grow through the challenges that we each face."

—Melinda Ribner
rabbinical pastor

Healing

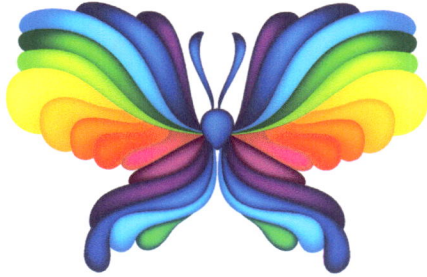

Healing

Cancer, Heart Disease, and Depression

Jerry Rhine
Survivor and Healer
Hopefulcare.com
Jerry@hopefulcare.com

Copyright © 2015 by Hopeful Care LLC

ISBN: 978-1-5040-2809-7

Distributed in 2015 by Open Road Distribution
345 Hudson Street
New York, NY 10014
www.openroadmedia.com

To my loving wife, Jennifer, who inspired me to survive and help others. Without her this book would never have been written and I would not be thriving.

To the following institutions which provided me with diagnosis and treatment:

Greenwich Hospital

Sloan Kettering

New York Presbyterian/ Weill Cornell Medical Center

Stamford Hospital

New York Medical Center

Burke Rehabilitation Hospital

And to M. D. Anderson for providing treatment for my brother so that 8 months after treatment there was no indication of the leukemia he had been diagnosed with.

Acknowledgments

This book is dedicated to the special heroes in my life:

Howard Anstendig, my beloved friend from age four to seventy-four was a giving man who bettered the lives of so many people. He will be fondly remembered by his patients, students, friends, and golf partners for his generous spirit. Howard courageously faced brain cancer for over a year, and will live in my heart forever.

Richard Mazer, my dear friend, who, during his five year battle with lymphoma shared with me that as long as he was with his wife Lynne, and could continue to make digital prints at his computer, he was happy.

Stephen Munzer, my dear friend from high school and college, who survived only six months after being diagnosed with non-Hodgkin's lymphoma, but who left his mark by making this world a better place just by having been in it.

Stephen Oster, my dear friend, who battled leukemia for five years and continued to be a leader at Chabad of Greenwich and in the Greenwich community.

Francine Port, my sister-in-law, who never permitted breast cancer to stop her from moving forward with her life and embracing her passion.

Donald Rhine, my brother, who in spite of medical pessimism, has overcome heart disease and advanced leukemia; and Michael Harris who lived with leukemia and was loved by every member of my family.

Imagery to Heal

The individuals reading this book, I expect, have either themselves or a member of their family has faced very difficult physical and emotional challenges in their lives. These people have
suffered from heart disease, cancer, emotional issues, and various other conditions. This presentation offers a way of coping
and empowering oneself in the face of these challenges. It is a
book about the subtle differences between healing and curing.
From my perspective, healing is defined as being able to lead
one's life complete with the positive emotions of joy, love, care,
and spirituality while still being able to express one's fears and
anger regarding the future. While *curing* is defined as ridding
oneself of the symptoms of psychological illness and physical
disease.

Imagery is a powerful tool of your imagination and sub-
conscious. Where cognitive therapy uses words, I use
imagery.

Images are constantly entering our minds both consciously and unconsciously in daydreams and night dreams.
The emotions inspired by these images affect which chemicals are received by our immune system and at what intensity.

Research studies have shown that imagery evoking positive emotions can change our negative mood and yield better
results and fewer side effects from medical treatment; it can

control the growth and metastasis of cancer cells and lessen the chance of recurrence. Imaging techniques greatly improve the quality of life of the survivor during and after treatment.

This presentation is not about me. I hope that the reader will observe me as a case study, lending credibility to the power of this work. This book is about each of you, your families, your friends, and your communities. As you look at the images contained in this book, I hope that you can try to personalize them with your own experiences. When possible, try to visualize the images in full by bringing in your other senses of hearing, touch, smell, and taste. Let the images bring back soothing and invigorating memories from you past or allow you to see positive events in the future. For memories, remember how you looked healthy and active, who you were with, smell the air around you, see the panorama surrounding you, hear the voices of friends or the sounds of nature, and remember what you were wearing at the time. Make the images as real as possible for you by individualizing the details. Sit back and enjoy. Remember, these visualizations are not meant to replace medical treatment when needed, but to enhance it and enable you to endure in the best possible manner.

Healing

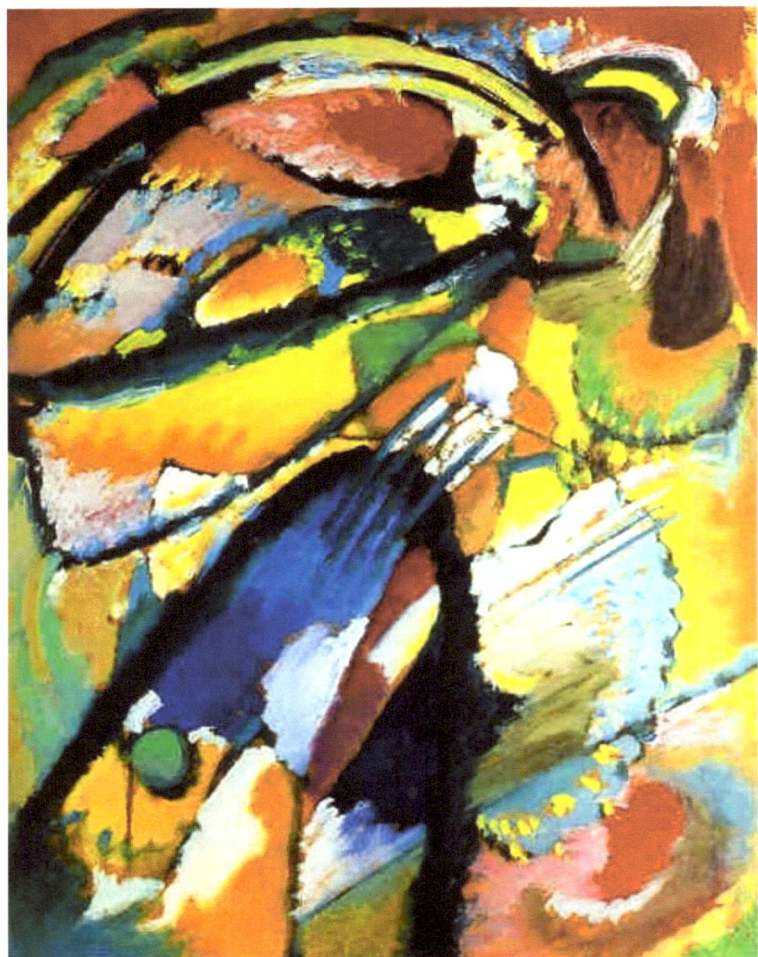

> ## "The world of reality has its limits; the world of imagination is boundless."
> *— Jean-Jacques Rousseau*

Imagine feeling positive emotions as you experience life-enforcing images. Create your own photograph, painting, sculpture, movie, or visual reality in your mind's eye. Bring in all your senses. Imagine smelling roses, hearing birds chirping, feeling the breeze on your skin, and tasting the salt water by an ocean beach. Imagine being in a forest, on a lake, in a place of worship, or above a cloud. Create in your mind's eye a calming, peaceful, protective place. It can be somewhere you visited in the past or somewhere you have always wanted to go. Bring in wise mentors like a grandmother, a teacher, a role model, a child, or a spiritual guide to help you to cope with your challenges. Using your intuition, explore potential solutions and their consequences. Learn what produces the best outcomes for you.

As the artistic director of your own images, you need to choose the palette, the textures, and the forms for your imagery. Pay attention to all of the details of the environment, including facial expressions and clothing. Watch what is happening, and listen to what is said.

Ponder now that you have done the exercise how does the imagery you visualized affect your thoughts and your emotions? The brain cannot distinguish between when you are imagining something and when you are actually experiencing it.

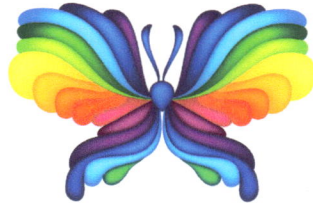

My experience: I imagine being at
a lake using all of my senses three times a day,
similar to the progressive relaxation
exercise at the end of the book.

Jerry Rhine

Change

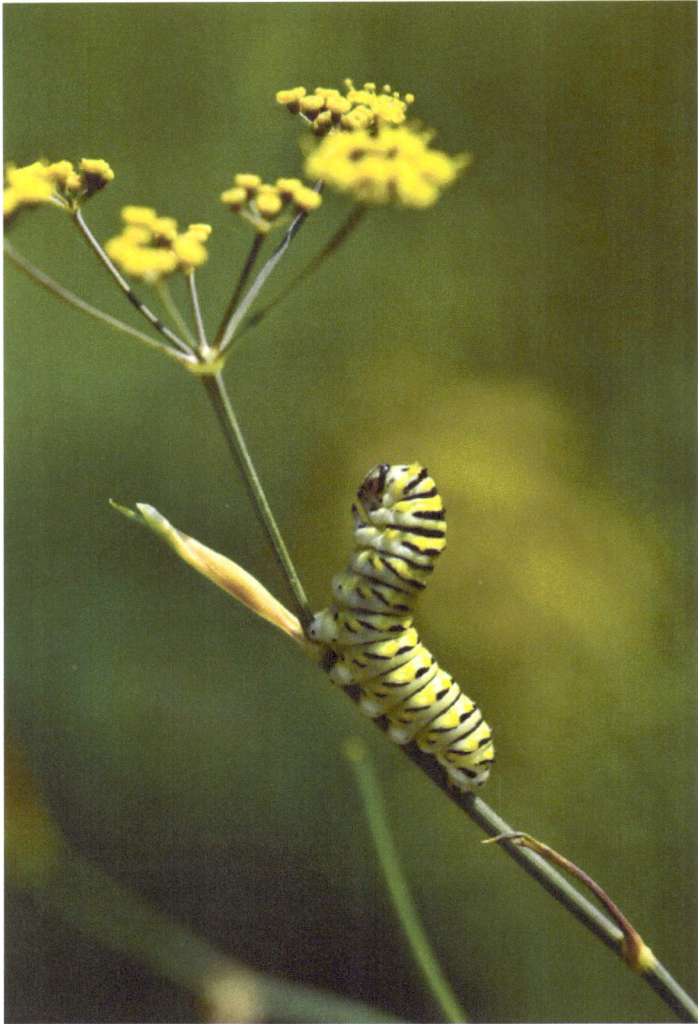

Change

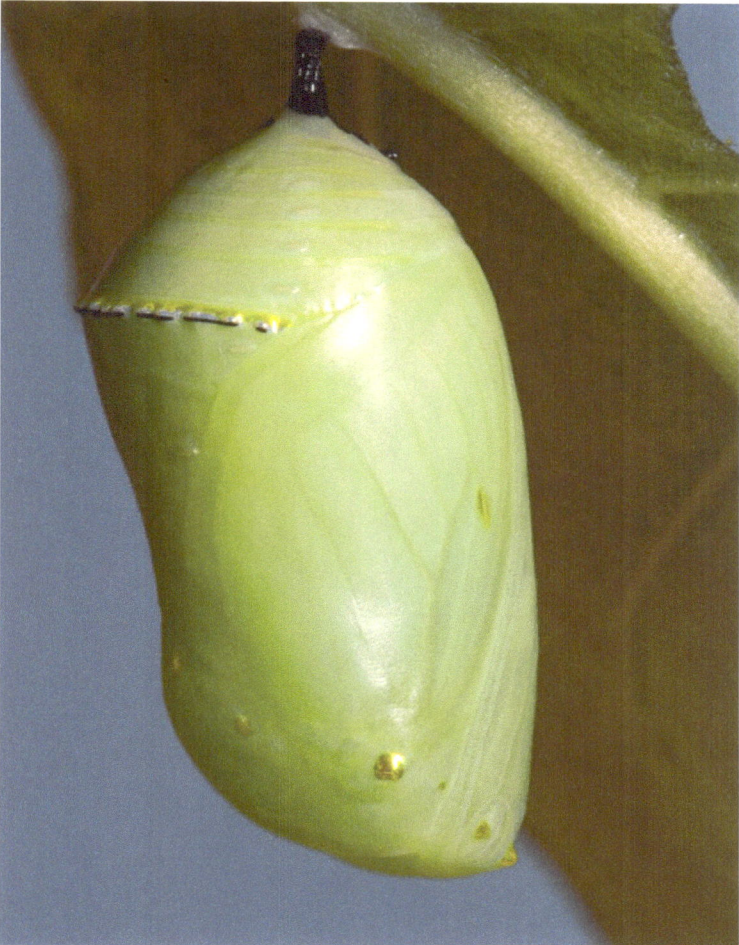

Jerry Rhine

Change

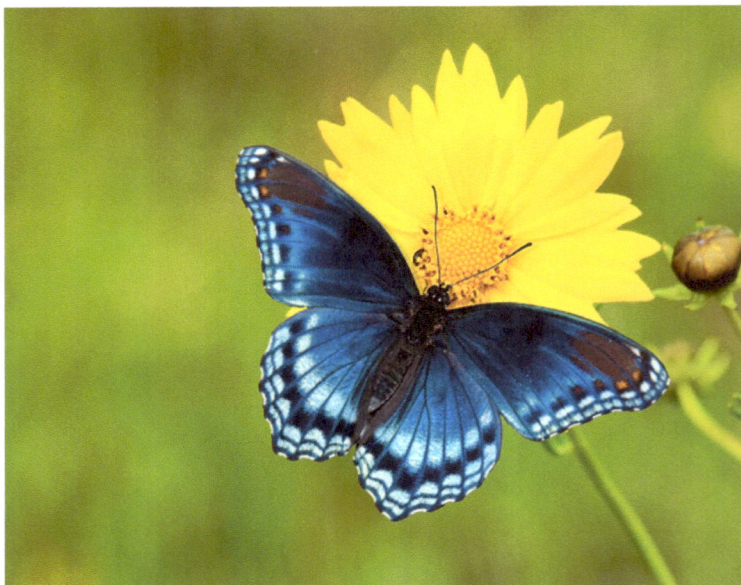

"The universe is change; our life is what our thoughts make it."
–Marcus Aurelius Antoninus

Imagine yourself in the future. See your body and soul becoming vibrant and healthy, and like a caterpillar; focus on nutrition, rest, and your metamorphosis. Imaging shedding your current illness as the caterpillar sheds its skin and your feelings of despair turn into hope and renewal. Know that you are encased in a protective cocoon while in this state of metamorphosis, which you will outgrow as your healing progresses.

Be introspective by seeking meaning and purpose in your life's journey. Empower yourself with spirituality to meet life's continuous challenges. Bring optimism into your life to extend longevity. Seek what you want to accomplish with the time remaining in your life be it six months or decades find what has interfered with your intentions. Learn what you can change in order to move toward your goals.

Allow yourself to be a butterfly—a beautiful part of nature. The word "butterfly" in ancient Greek is ψυχή *(psȳchē)*, which means "soul/mind." The butterfly signifies rebirth, resurrection, celebration, lightness, freedom, time, soul, joyous times, and love. The rebirth that is healing is possible because of the mind-body connection that has been recognized since the time of Aristotle.

Initially, we feel impotent to change the outcome of illness, and this leads to hopelessness. We are not helpless; we are partners with our doctors, alternative healers, therapists, and caregivers. We can empower our minds and souls to strengthen our immune system and ultimately reverse illness.

Ponder that living things in stasis die. Our lives are not static, but constantly changing. Given ongoing environmental challenges and burdens, we are continuously seeking homeostasis. We frequently adapt by changing our thoughts and moods, which influence the chemicals in our bodies. Our cells are changing, dying and recreating, while receiving new information. Our immune system either activates or moderates and, in turn, acts to implode cancer cells and return to a state of harmony.

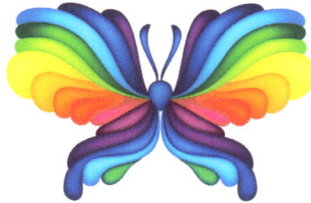

My experience: I felt as if I was a burden on my family and was contributing nothing. I felt that there was no reason to get out of bed in the morning. I sought help from a psychiatrist and a rabbi, which culminated in my traveling to Israel for guidance and help. I changed from a real estate broker to a social worker and a certified Jewish healer to help others overcome challenges similar to mine.

Jerry Rhine

Hope

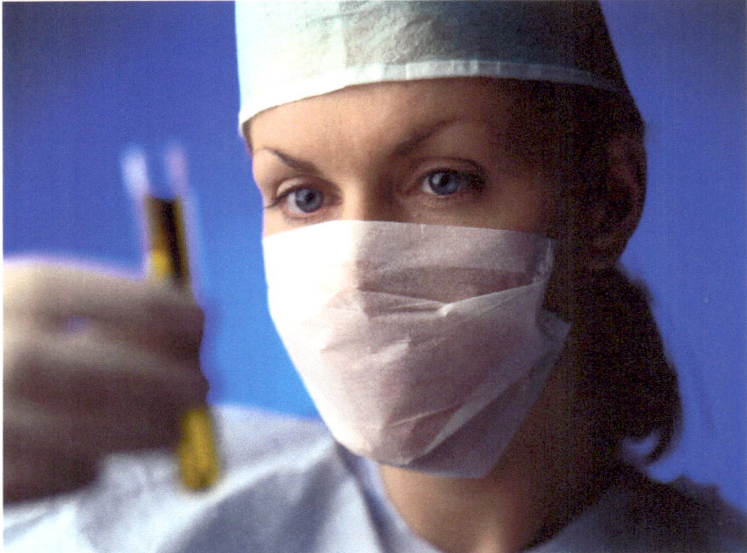

"I find hope in the darkest of days, and focus in the brightest. I do not judge the universe."
–Dalai Lama

Imagine the hope of healing. See yourself through imaging as thriving, achieving, giving and helping to create a better universe and world for you and those you love. Allow yourself to hear your strong inner voice.

Our expectations have a profound effect on how we heal. Studies show that the information the brain expects to receive in the near future affects the physical state of the body. This means that hope and positive thoughts are essential for survival: patients who think positively recover better from chronic illnesses since they are active participants in their recovery and not passive victims. Since thoughts and emotions influence physical well-being, taking care of your spirit is just as important as taking care of your body to recover from an illness.

Ponder that I was told in 2004 that I had months to live. My cancer had progressed to stage three, and then my cancer stopped spreading and the tumors ceased growing. Science and miracles go hand in hand.

Remember that the longer you live, the greater the chance that a cure will be found in your lifetime. Laboratories and hospitals are exploring new drugs and procedures for heart disease, cancer and more.

Clinical trials are creating breakthroughs everyday. Even though there is a long way to go, the progress that has been made in the past decade is impressive and promising.

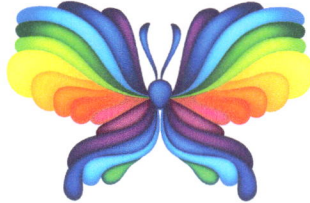

My experience: In the 1980s, I met Robert Good, a top researcher who believed the immune system was the key to finding a cure for cancer. As a pioneer in the study of stem cell research that continues today, he was featured on the cover of *Time Magazine*.

The *New York Times* reported in 2011 that gene therapy was used to enhance T cells, a type of white cell in the immune system that kills cancer cells and can eliminate cancer in a patient. In 2013, the University of Pennsylvania reported using gene therapy for leukemia patients resulting in complete remission in some cases.

Jerry Rhine

Knowledge

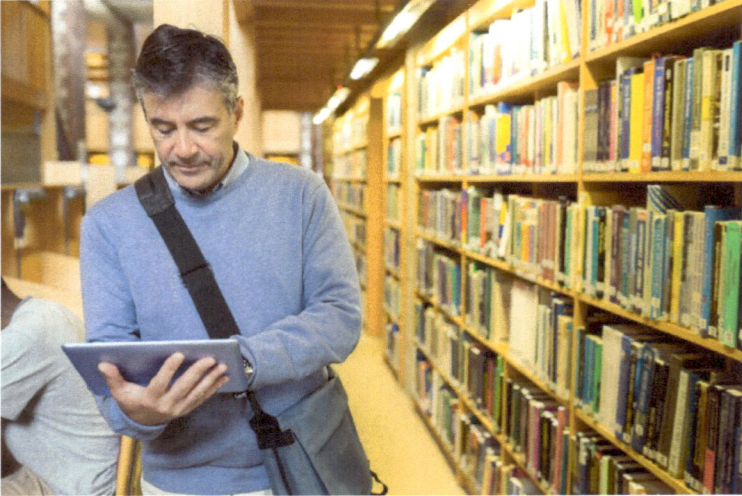

"All our knowledge has its origins in our perceptions."
– *Leonardo da Vinci*

Imagine learning new things. Let your mind be open and explore new possibilities. Like a student, find lessons you can apply to your life. Recapture the curiosity you had as a child. Seek out information about alternative medicines and therapies that might help you. Learn what laboratories are conducting research focused on the type of illness that you are dealing with. Be open-minded in considering your treatment options. See potential solutions from different perspectives. Investigate alternative strategies about altering your brain and body to reverse disease. Challenge the norm and decide what the truth is for you. Seek to know if there is a personal meaning to your disease. Learn what is creating conflict and distress in your life. Let knowledge empower you and allay your fear.

Ponder the nature of your illness and seek to understand it so that you can partner with your doctors and other caregivers to achieve change and enhance your ability to heal.

Jerry Rhine

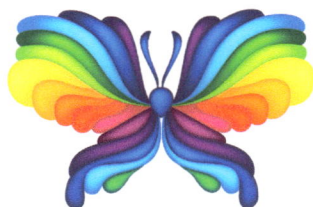

My experience: I traveled to Jerusalem to meet with Rabbis and healers in order to learn new strategies, including how to imagine a direct connection to God's presence and how to visualize positive past events and see positive events in the future. According to the testing that was done on me at Sloan Kettering Hospital in New York City, after my diagnosis and before I began medical treatment, the size of my cancer tumor had reduced by more than fi fty percent. At age sixty-seven, I went to New York University to get my master's degree in social work. I subsequently received certification as a spiritual healer. I acquired the knowledge to help others and to heal myself.

Self-Love

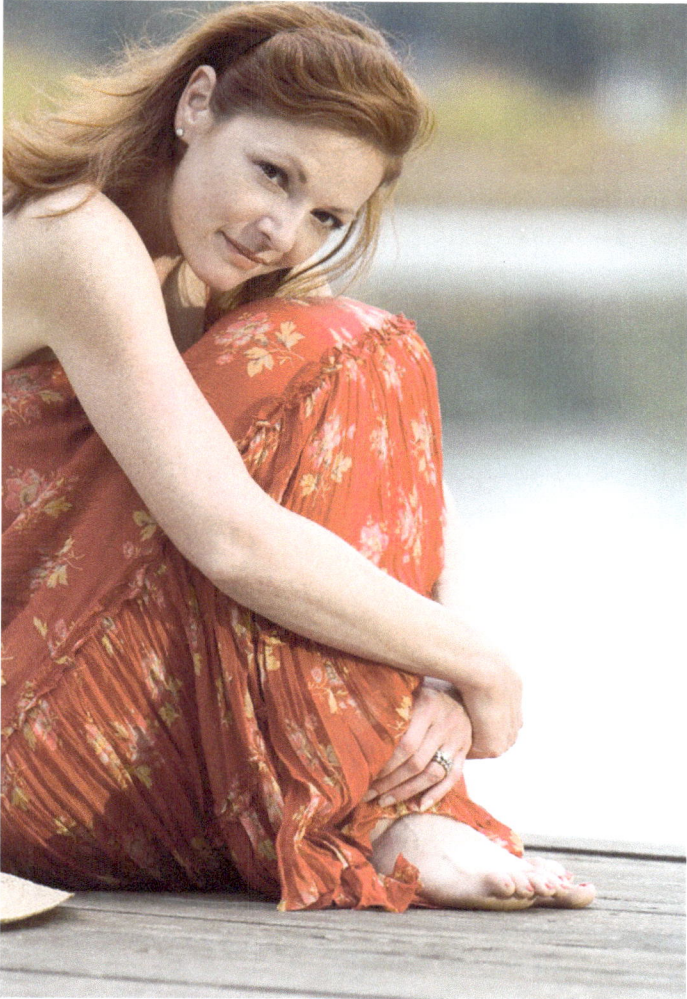

"Self-love is the source of all our other loves."
– *Pierre Corneille*

Imagine giving yourself a comforting hug. Let your body become calm and infused with caring thoughts. Find acceptance that you are doing your best, given your challenges, genes, and environment. Don't allow self-hatred to block your ability to heal. Let self-love bring the positive results of a better mood and possibly much more. Love yourself unconditionally. Take steps to fulfill your purpose.

Ponder that some of us, like myself, may not have been given the love we needed from a parent who experienced the same deprivation from his or her parent, but did his or her very best. This lack of love from others may result in unreasonable guilt and self-blame, which may get in the way of self-love. Be aware, and change through visualization these kinds of thoughts, which affect your mood and health both negatively both consciously and unconsciously.

Given genetic makeup and challenging life events such as the loss of a spouse, an economic downturn, a divorce, or the loss of a job, we do not always have it in our power to prevent chronic disease and chronic pain. Like a hurricane, a natural event, they just happen. What in your life is creating great conflict and distress?

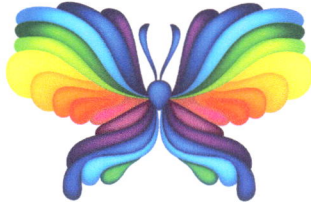

My experience: My purpose is to teach others the strategies that have healed me in mind body and spirit. I've worked with people to help them identify their strengths, which are empowering, instead of ruminating about their weaknesses, which are self-defeating.

Jerry Rhine

Happiness

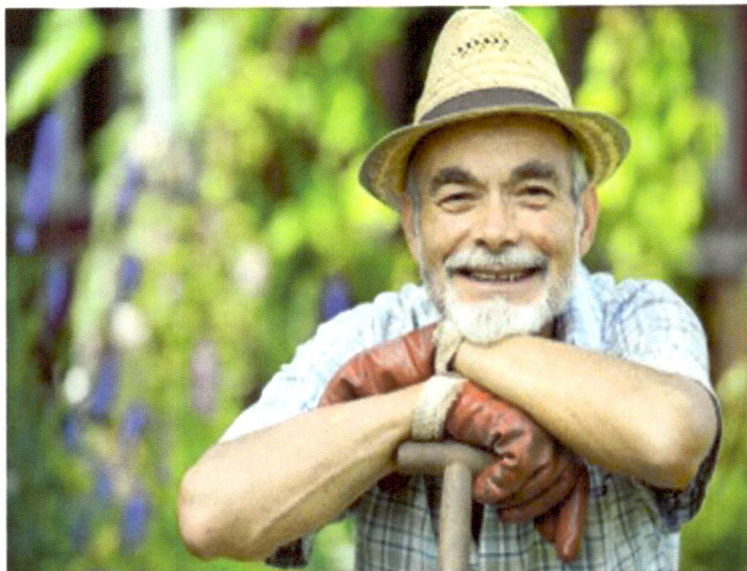

> "Happiness is spiritual, born of truth and love. It is unselfish; therefore it cannot exist alone, but requires all mankind to share it."
> *– Mary Baker Eddy*

Imagine trust, kindness, and compassion. Let your body feel the embrace of one who cares for you.

Ponder that Dean Ornish, MD, was a pioneer in alternative medicine. In his book, *Love & Survival*, he outlines the scientific basis for the healing power of intimacy. He states that love and intimacy are at the root of what makes us sick and what makes us well, what causes sadness and what brings happiness, what causes suffering and what causes healing. He talks of emotional and spiritual disease caused by profound feelings of loneliness, isolation, anger, hostility, cynicism, alienation, and depression.

Dean Ornish states that in addition to someone at home whom you appreciate, lean on, feel close to, can be vulnerable with, share feelings with, and confide in, a community can provide social support to meet many of your essential emotional needs. If these needs are not met, studies show that you will have a three to five times higher risk of premature death and disease. Your immune system is less effective when you are in conflict with your spouse or companion. Some cancer survivors like me have been isolated because of the stigma associated with the disease.

Many so-called friends disappear not knowing how to relate now that you have a life-threatening illness. Studies by Dr. Spiegel have shown that support from group therapy is particularly beneficial to cancer patients. You benefit from the empathy of others; you feel empowered by empathizing with others. Sharing experiences removes some of the stigma of disease. You can fulfill your psychosocial needs in a variety of ways. We have the potential to enrich each other's lives as we meet the challenges of interpersonal relationships.

Quantum physics, which deals with the smallest particles, demonstrates how change in a particle can influence change in another particle one mile away. Our consciousness affects the behavior of subatomic particles, which in turn alters our cells. We all have the ability to change and be changed by loving and being loved by others. Confine toxic people and unpleasant thoughts to a bubble and let them float away into the sky.

There are over forty Happiness Clubs coast to coast as well as happiness clubs throughout the world. According to Lionel Ketchian founder of the Happiness Club, "You can be Happy right now and for every moment to come for the rest of your life. Being Happy is the most powerful skill you can learn. Being in the present moment is essential to happiness. Awareness is a critical ingredient of happiness.

Most of our thinking is about obsessing over things we have no control over. Happiness is a way to inner peace and an inner state of well being that enables you to profit from your highest thoughts, intelligence, wisdom, awareness, common sense, health, and spiritual values." Go to HappinessClub.com to find a club near you. There are Happiness Clubs in Israel, Jordan, France, Switzerland, India, Pakistan, and Hong Kong as well.

Jerry Rhine

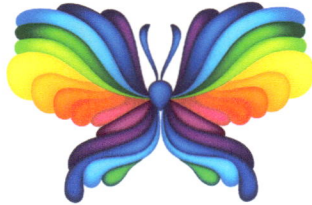

My experience: I spent a day with Dean Ornish, and my recovery from advanced heart disease has been miraculous. He lectured on the effectiveness of diet, humor, relaxation techniques and intimacy in altering the narrowing of your arteries. He made me feel hopeful that I would be able to reverse my heart disease. A diet of less than 20% fat has contributed to the strengthening my heart. Ensuring I am surrounded by humorous and uplifting people, making emotional meaningful connections with members of Chabad, and visualizations have all contributed to my recovery. I have been an ambassador based in Fairfield County, CT of Happiness Clubs.

Self-Esteem

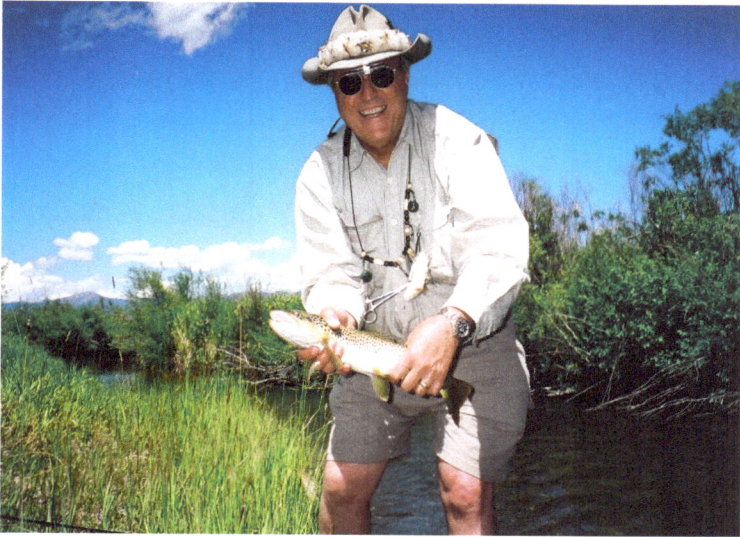

> **"Self-esteem is as important to our well-being as legs are to a table. It is essential for physical and mental health and for happiness."**
>
> *– Louise Hart*

Imagine overcoming an insurmountable challenge and standing on the top of a mountain. Create a film like *It's a Wonderful Life* in your mind featuring the major events you are most proud of. Focus on the stories of those whom you have helped. Portray the overwhelming challenges in your life that you have survived. See your major accomplishments and what you have nurtured or created. As a director, pay attention to detail and make it as real as possible.

If you experience the loss of self-esteem with illness, return to old passions or develop new ones. Do crafts, play a musical instrument, try fly-fishing, or do photography to record your family's events. Explore your talents to enrich your life and improve your feelings about yourself.

Ponder that chronic illness can result in the loss of function and capabilities. In some cases, you become dependent on others or have to reinvent yourself.

Changes in your body from treatment can greatly affect your self-image.

Men treated for prostate cancer often experience impotence and incontinence for various periods of time that make them feel emotionally inadequate. Women who have under-gone mastectomies experience a change in their feelings about their bodies and sexual attractiveness. It is critical at these times to look to your strengths. Often chronic illness arises after retirement and after children have left the nest. These events can also affect your self-image.

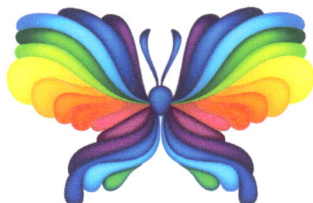

My Experience: I lost my long-standing, lucrative career as a commercial real estate broker and had to depend on my wife's income to support not just me, but our entire family. I became a social worker and a spiritual healer to maintain my self-esteem, and feel that I had returned to being a contributing member of society and to my family. Unfortunately, I developed non-Hodgkin's lymphoma shortly after graduating from NYU.

Courage

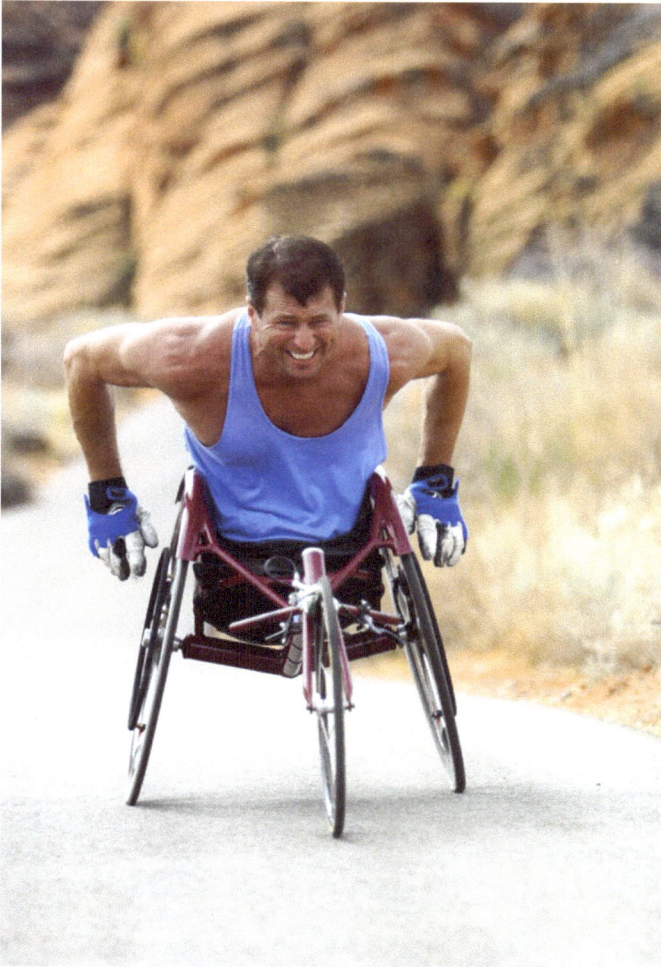

> ## "We gain strength, and courage, and confidence by each experience in which we really stop to look fear in the face ... we must do that which we think we cannot."
> *—Eleanor Roosevelt*

Affirmation for Courage

"My radiantly positive thoughts impart hope, joy, and courage."

—Sheilla Randall

Imagine yourself confronting danger and living through it. Imagine your immune system and the treatments you are receiving encircling and destroying cancerous tumors by cutting off the chemicals the tumor needs to survive. Imagine a healthy you at peace in the future.

Create a movie that takes place at an earlier time in your life when you faced what seemed to be an insurmountable challenge. In making your movie you need to consider the following:

How did you overcome this obstacle?

Where and when did this event occur?

What were your emotions at the time that you faced the obstacle that you thought was insurmountable?

Who was involved in either causing the problem or helping you create a solution?

What were these characters like?

What were the details?

Make sure your costume designer gets it right. Make the scenery real. This movie should involve all the senses, including smell and touch. It can be like virtual reality.

You could also create in your mind a video where you are the captain of a boat that is tossing around in an uncontrollable manner in a major storm with ten-foot waves and violent winds. Imagine you are guiding the boat through the turbulence, without panic, all the while circumventing the many obstacles in your path that you cannot control. Navigate your way to calmer peaceful waters at the end of the journey.

Whenever I underwent medical tests, I had more courage than I had imagined I would. Since my initial cancer metastasized, the resulting treatments caused me great discomfort, making me barely able to function and take care of my own physical needs. There were times when the pain was so great, I would scream out in the middle of the night and had to use oxycodone as well as fentanyl, both of which are highly addictive opiates, like heroin. Fortunately, despite alcoholism in my twenties, using prayer and visualization, I did not become addicted.

Ponder that we have the ability to confront fear, danger, and uncertainty in the face of physical pain, hardship, or threat of death. Cancer can feel like a battlefield. It is a personal journey that one must sometimes undertake without the help of others. We are alone in our thoughts, but we don't have to be. Still, we can be role models, and we can hope that others come to see disease as only a part of themselves and overcome adversity.

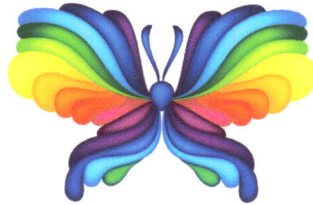

My experience: The tumor on my spine progressed to the point that I had to use a cane and ultimately a walker in order to safely navigate on my own. I was unable to drive a car due to the narcotics that I was required to take to combat the constant pain. Living in the suburbs without public transportation, I became dependent on others for going to doctor's appointments, to temple, shopping, and seeing friends. I became withdrawn and the loss of independence for someone who was used to working and traveling independently and playing golf was impossible to accept. I became angry and, in retrospect, I realized that as my emotional state of mind deteriorated so did my physical ability to function and ambulate. I had to consciously force myself to step back from my current state of health and look at the bigger picture that included the treatments working, my health improving, my ability to regain my physical and emotional strength, and my connection to those around me returning. I refused to allow myself to be defeated. I have put my efforts into speaking, writing, and teaching so that I can give people hope by sharing my own experiences. I now drive again, play golf every weekend and, after throwing away the unused narcotics, have donated my walker and cane to Goodwill.

Freedom

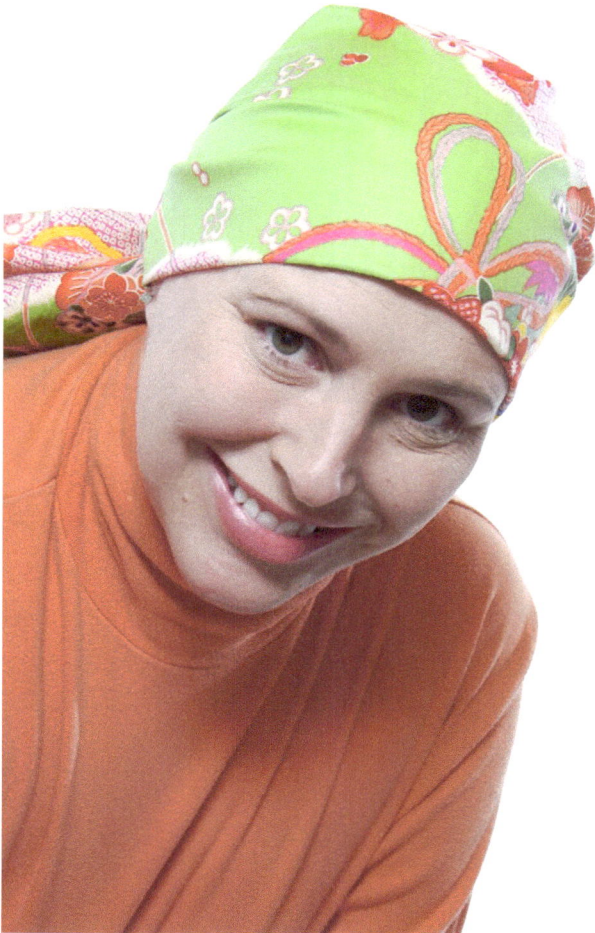

"Freedom is what you do with what's been done to you."
– *Jean-Paul Sartre*

Affirmation for Freedom

"Every day I am getting closer to total **freedom**. Every day I become more spontaneous and playful. Every day I create the feeling of unlimited **freedom** in my life."

—Che Garmin

Imagine doing dangerous things that you passionately wanted to do, but did not have the nerve. Choose to climb a mountain, drive a racing car, or explore the depths of an ocean.

Let the fear that the awareness of your mortality has brought you lead to increased freedom. Allow the restraints put on us by family and society become insignificant. Be more authentic and don't hide who you really are to please others.

Please yourself. Loosen your chains and explore your dreams about what you want to experience in life. Try to fulfill your dreams and fantasies. Be stimulated or thrilled according to your individual needs.

Ponder that if you are a woman who has lost her hair from chemotherapy, choose scarves of many beautiful colors and designs. Acknowledge that this may be a time of great discomfort and you deserve to pamper yourself. Create your own fashion statement as a survivor. Go shopping. Buy shoes, jewelry, or dresses in bolder colors and designs. Put on makeup that will make you feel better about yourself. Take advantage of the chance to express your unique self. Go to the movies, theatre, or a nightclub with your girlfriends. Get your nails done, a massage, or a facial. Try things new for you or things you have not done in a long time like reading a trashy novel, learning to tango, or going to a bird sanctuary. The world is open to your imagination. Feel childlike or somewhat irresponsible, letting others take care of your chores without guilt. Plan a trip with a close girlfriend. Bonding and sharing intimate information can help your emotional health. Have dark chocolate, a latte, and eat a decadent desert. Take a bubble bath, play country, baroque classical music, or whatever music may comfort you. Light a candle with a soothing scent. Drink a glass of wine or the milkshake that you always thought was too fattening. Pull a comforter over you while watching old movies on Hulu or Netflix. Men can take a hot bath playing jazz or whatever sooths them. Drink a bottle of Guinness stout. Buy a bright belt or suspenders. Grow a beard or change the style of your hair. Men and women can free themselves and enjoy some of the things that are traditionally thought of as connected to the other gender. As I said earlier, humor is a great distraction. Watch your favorite comic, which might be Johnny Carson or whoever you favor.

At some point you can accept the inevitable in a positive way. Write or record a book stating all the wonderful things you did in your life to make this a better world. They may be basic things like helping a friend or relative. Use your imagination to do the unique. A father of 62 with stage 4 pancreatic cancer, and just months to live, wanted to do something special for his young daughter since he knew he would not be alive when she was a bride. He arranged for his young daughter to get a beautiful wedding dress, and for a wedding ceremony pronouncing them "Daddy and Daughter." Proudly, he walked her down the aisle giving her a wonderful memory.

Another father wrote over 800 notes, which could be put in his daughter's lunchbox until she graduated high school.

A woman with cancer of the bowels, which spread to liver, lungs, and pelvis, wrote a book called *Humor with a Tumor*. She spoke of the support she received from her husband, and said that while being diagnosed with cancer was scary it does not have to defi ne you. She wrote birthday cards for her son through his 21st birthday.

Movies have depicted wonderful resistance to cancer. In *The Bucket List* a corporate billionaire and a working-class mechanic have only their cancer in common. They decide to do all those things that they always dreamed of doing, but were prevented by practicality or suspected danger. In the process, they become very close friends and found joy in life. You must have the experiences you dreamed of doing but rejected or said "someday." Now may be the time. In a film called *Step Mom*, Anna is diagnosed with lymphoma and gives her daughter a beautiful quilt with family photos and memorabilia such as her first step and the horse her daughter rode on stitched in. Maybe you can create a collage, photo albums, or maybe even a quilt. My wife has made many wonderful photo albums of family events. Looking at them brings back wonderful family memories, which ease the challenges of the present.

Jerry Rhine

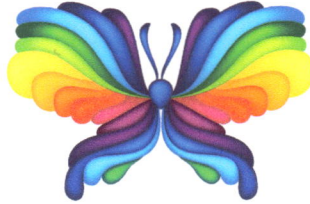

My experience: Against the advice of social workers who were concerned I would fail and fall into a deep depression, I started graduate school at age sixty-seven and succeeded in earning a master's degree in social work. Getting through the frustration connected with academic work made me feel more self-confident, and utilizing the disability accommodations available to me at New York University made it possible for me to reach my potential. During the summers, I traveled to Costa Rica and later to Guatemala, improving my Spanish while living with struggling families. I learned to dance the salsa, lived on a meager diet compared to that in the USA which lead to my losing weight and experiencing a very different culture filled with deep faith and a real closeness with three generations each taking care of the other. I met people from the United States and many young

young people from Germany who had also come to volunteer and help. While there, I dyed my white hair brown, but it looked like a terrible mop. I tried.

Jerry Rhine

Compassion

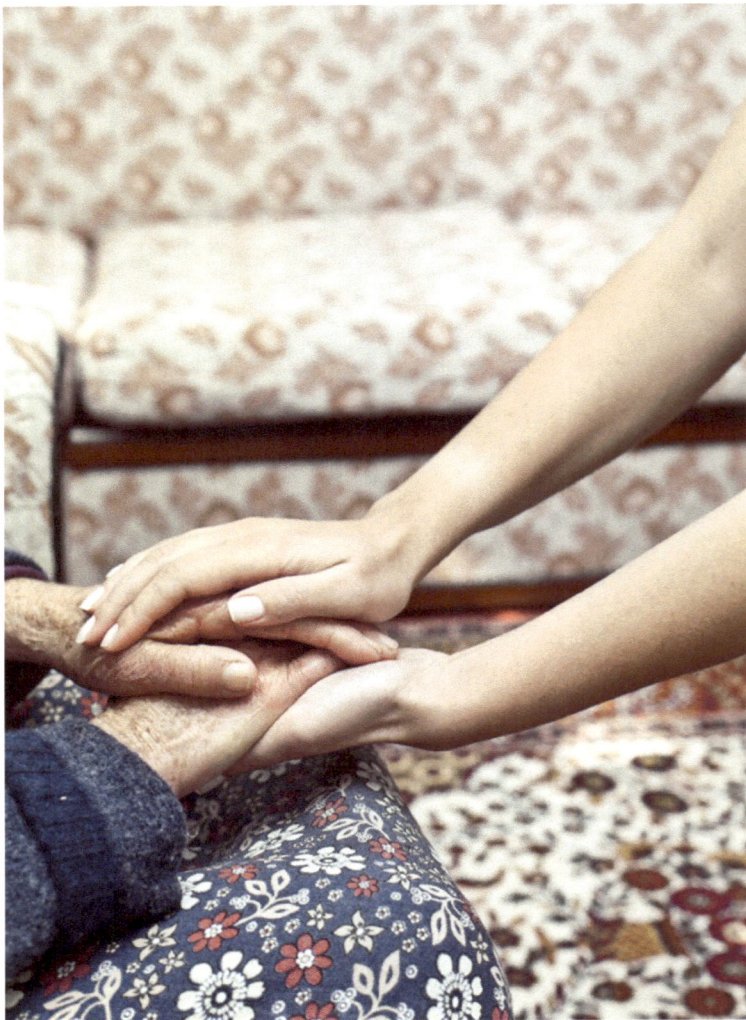

> ## "But my experience is that people who have been through painful, difficult times are filled with compassion."
> *—Amy Grant*

Imagine yourself and your friends and family woven into a blanket of compassion. Choose a compassionate primary doctor who understands your suffering and can interface on your behalf with the specialists who will be retained to assist with your recovery. It is critical that you have a compassionate primary physician who can quarterback your treatment, explain the medical jargon that others use when talking to you, interpret the myriad of tests and results, recommend options and coordinate the services that you are going to need beyond doctors.

It's important to surround yourself with positive influences, so consider taking a step back from toxic people who minimize the importance of your illness and are scared of their own vulnerability. You will be shocked by casual acquaintances who come forward with an outstretched hand and offer support. Try and be present for others even if you can do no more than listen and ask them whether you can help. Help them focus on their inner well-being and walk in another's shoes.

Ponder that others with cancer and heart disease are suffering just like you. You can support each other with compassion as you share each other's experiences.

Join support groups. Contact other survivors. Feel the positive emotions that will bring you happiness and change the chemicals in your body.

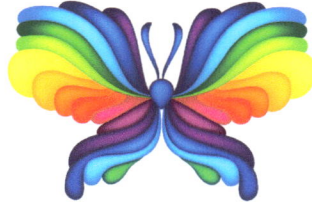

My experience: My first oncologist and cardiologist temporarily eliminated my hope and my wife's by telling us I had a short time to live. A psychiatrist told me I was a shirker when my brain damage confined me to working on an assembly line according to two days of psychosocial testing. Thankfully, I found competent, compassionate doctors who lessened my fear. My neurologist always said I was a miracle. I have shown compassion by helping people who are blind and engaging in conversation on busses with isolated people in wheelchairs. I received smiles and tears and left with a feeling of joy.

Jerry Rhine

Power

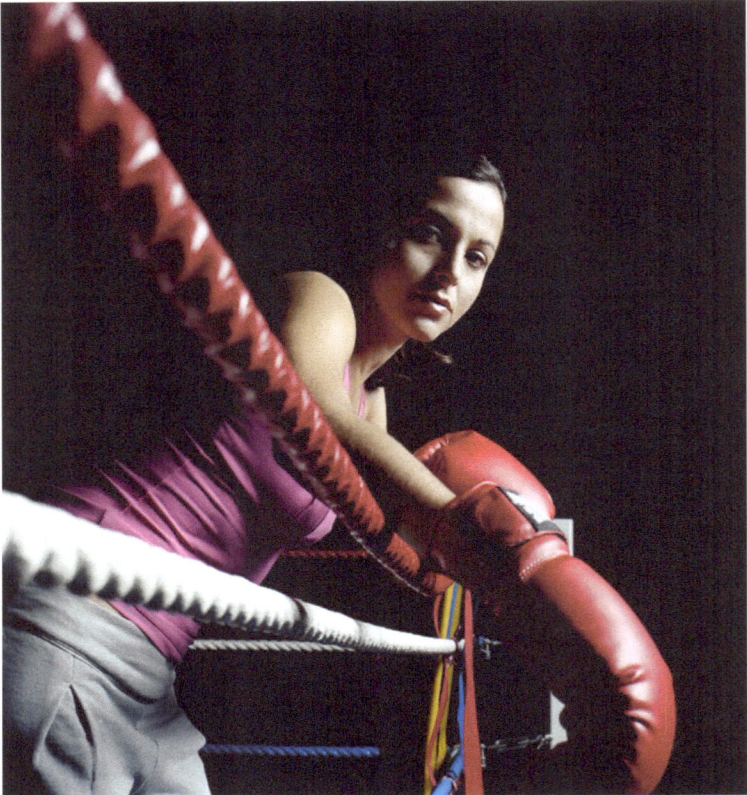

"What it lies in our power to do, it lies in our power not to do."
—Aristotle

Imagine the power within you. Your immune system is a natural fighter you need to keep at peak performance. Control and change your thoughts to benefit yourself.

Ponder that the mind generates a constant flow of thoughts (an average of sixty thousand per day) out of which more than ninety percent are habitual or conditioned thoughts.

Cancer cannot take away our positive emotions. It is our choice to express them. You can keep positive throughout sixty thousand thoughts if you do so consciously, and try using some of the techniques in this book. Visualize in order to change.

We almost always have the power to determine how we react to our thoughts when we choose to react positively. This may lead to a better outcome.

Victor Frankl, a scientist and psychiatrist, survived the concentration camp at Auschwitz during World War II. While at Sloan Kettering during a research study on the effect of spirituality on cancer patients, a social worker gave me Frankl's book, *Man's Search for Meaning*. Frankl believed that survival depended less on illness and age than on having a sense of meaning. He credits his survival at the concentration camp to thoughts and images of his wife. His wife had already been murdered and cremated in the camp, but he still imagined her loving embrace. Frankl also visualized completing his scientific work after he was freed from the camp.

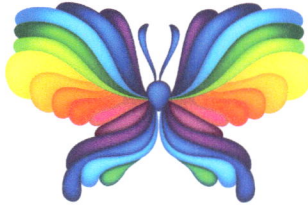

My experience: Aiding others is empowering.
I receive power from helping others with
cancer, heart disease, and other afflictions.

Jerry Rhine

Joy

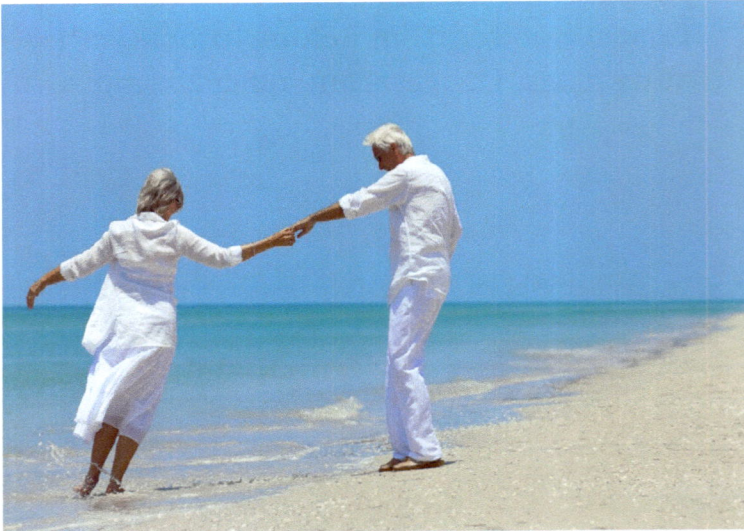

> **"We are shaped by our thoughts; we become what we think. When the mind is pure, joy follows like a shadow that never leaves."**
> *– Buddha*

Affirmation for Joy

"I see the beauty in my surroundings and I radiate joy and love."

"I am grateful for all the wonderful things I already have in my life and those that are yet to come."

"Joy is in my heart and in my life. I project It to everyone I interact with. I choose to be joyful."

—Dornea Horn

Imagine that you have achieved your desires and overcome your limitations. Find pleasure in everyday experiences, delight in small feats, and meet the challenges cancer has presented to you.

Ponder that joy can change the biochemical transmitters in your body and heal you. These include serotonin, endorphins, and dopamine.

Jerry Rhine

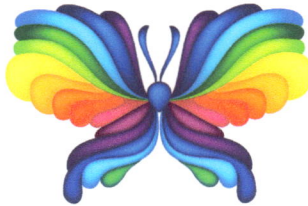

My experience: I find joy in the accomplishments of my family and friends. Twenty years ago when I first became ill, I could not imagine being alive to be at my children's bar and bat mitzvahs, but I was present, not just at those ceremonies, but at their graduations from high school and first days in college. Visualizing their futures and dreaming about my presence at their graduations from college, weddings, as well as their having successful careers, brings me joy, which aids in my healing.

Laughter

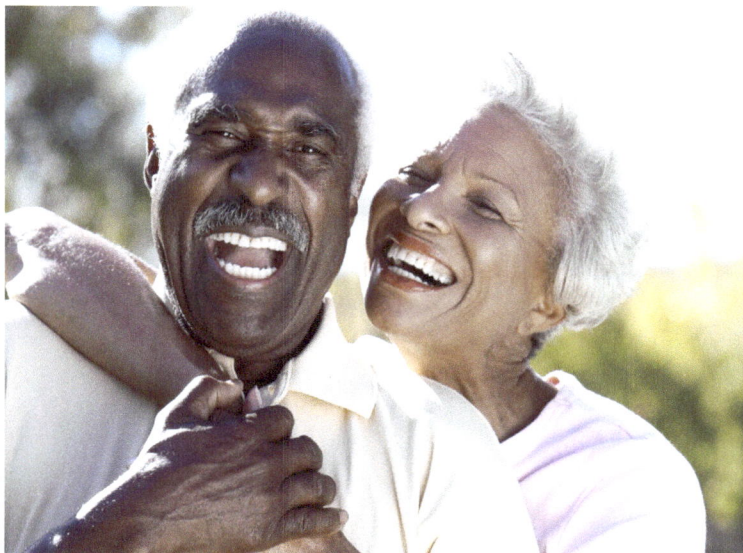

"Comedy is defiance. It's a snort of contempt in the face of fear and anxiety. And it's the laughter that allows hope to creep back on the inhale."
—Will Durst

Imagine something funny that makes your belly shake with laughter. When you laugh, you create healthy chemical changes in your body by producing serotonin. Watch your favorite comedians on YouTube or on DVD. Go to comedy-cures.com to find jokes for those dealing with cancer.

I had survived more than ten years after an oncologist told my wife and me that I had a short time to live. I felt like Truman after the election, holding up a newspaper that said "Dewey Wins." You can laugh at the unpredictability of life. Anything is possible, including recovery. Laugh at those who do not know of your inner strength, love, and faith.

Ponder that Norman Cousins, famous for his work on positive thinking, used humor therapy. Cousins had cancer, but with the consent of his doctors, he checked himself out of the hospital and into a hotel across the street.

He invited friends over and watched a lot of comedy fi lms and laughed a lot! He discovered that laughter relieves pain and helps heal cancer.

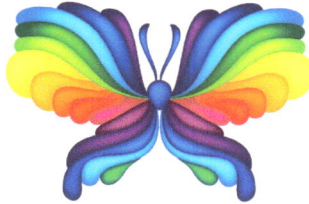

My experience: As part of my Non-Hodgkin's Lymphoma, I had an inoperable tumor resting on my spinal cord. It caused excruciating pain until the combination of radiation, chemotherapy and imaging reduced the size of the tumor and resulting pressure on my spinal cord. Oxycodone and comedy helped me cope; comedy made me feel better and imagine a world beyond myself.

I attended a program for cancer patients at Greenwich Hospital, near where I live. The speaker espoused the wonderful benefits of comedy. Though I consider myself an intellectual lover of Bach and German Expressionist art, I started watching and enjoying slapstick films featuring Charlie Chaplin, The Three Stooges, Milton Berle, Jerry Lewis, and Lucille Ball.

Jerry Rhine

Awe

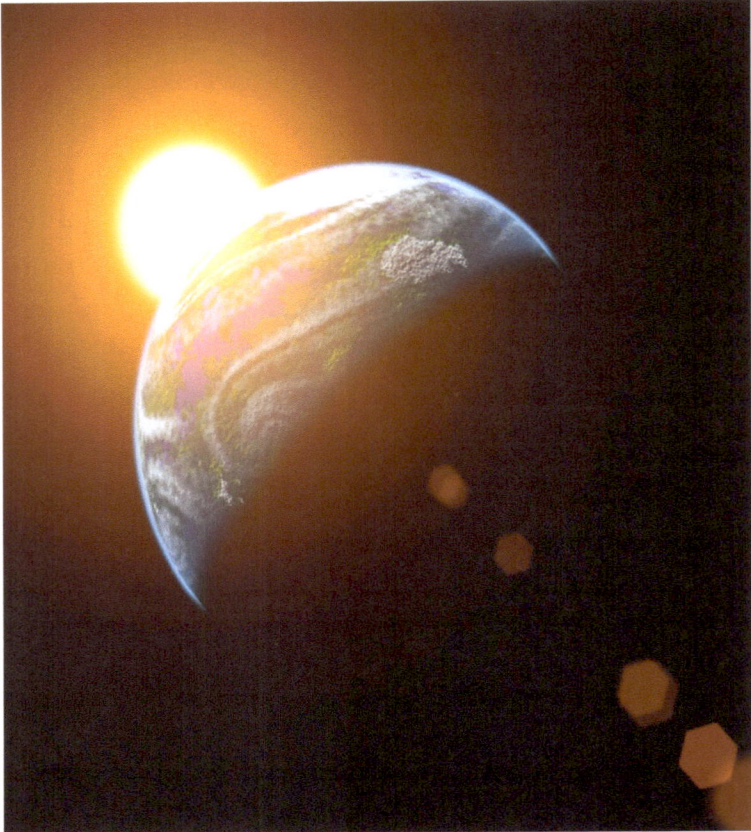

"I stand in awe of my body."
– Henry David Thoreau

Affirmation for Awe

"I stand in Awe. The infinite and eternal universe is my foundation and source. I stand in Awe. In Joy."

—Cherl Trine

Imagine yourself filled with awe. Ponder the incredible anatomy of your body and see the natural systems that protect you from cancer. See the inside of your magnificent brain and body in action. See the cells, neurotransmitters, and hormone that are communicating signals to heal you.

Ponder that when something dangerous happens in our environment and creates emotions of fear and anxiety, the body releases hormones, including cortisol and epinephrine, from our adrenal glands.

This stress response is protective in the short run, but if intensely active over time, it is destructive to the immune system. Overwhelming stress can occur when we experience traumas such as cancer or heart disease. Long-term stress from divorce, unemployment, or isolation can cause the body to release these stress hormones. Another hormone called serotonin, which is produced when we are happy, can positively enhance the immune system. We release this hormone with positive experiences.

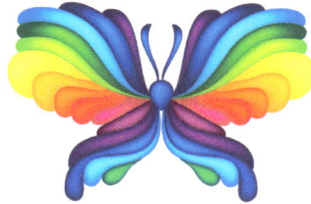

My experience: I am in awe of how visualization allowed my immune system to shrink a tumor over fifty percent according to testing done at Sloan Kettering Hospital in New York City.

Jerry Rhine

Gratitude

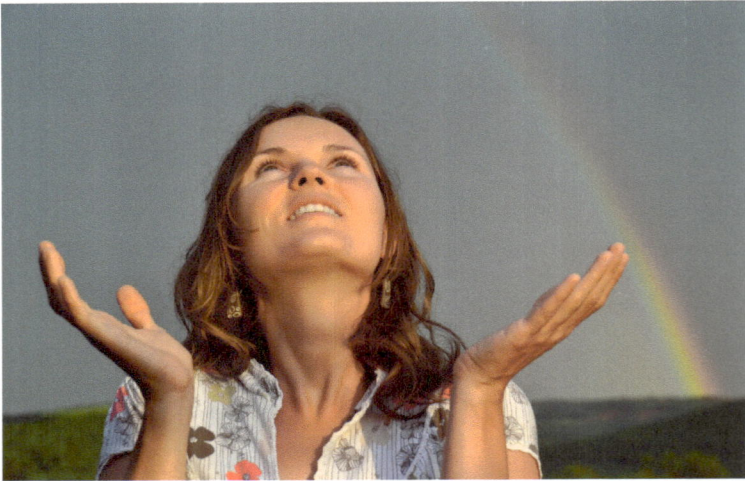

"Gratitude changes the pangs of memory into tranquil joy."
—Dietrich Bonhoeffer

Imagine the blessings you have received. Through the pain of life, acknowledge the happiness. Appreciate family, friends, community, and nature, which come to you freely. Rather than focusing on what you can't do, focus on what you can do, no matter how simple it is. Rather than being arrogant or greedy by taking things for granted and feeling entitled to all you desire, be thankful for memories of beautiful experiences.

Ponder that gratitude is an important part of spirituality and helps us find inner peace. It is a healing agent for our body and a healing energy in our lives.

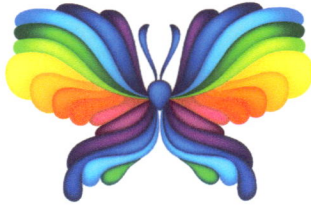

My experience: While a tumor rested on my
esophagus, I screamed out at the dinner
table and scared my family, especially
my young children.
The chronic pain had restricted what
I was able to do, including driving and interacting in
a meaningful way with my children. They needed an
active parent who could be emotionally and
physically present in their lives. In addition, as part
of my treatment for prostate cancer, I had
radioactive pellets inserted in my prostate
and, as a result, I had to be at least 20 feet
away from my children at all times in order to
protect them. How do you explain to an 8 year old
why you cannot read next to them in bed, cuddle on
the couch or help them with their homework?

I could not even go out in public out of fear of
encountering a pregnant woman and putting her
unborn baby at risk. I became more isolated, though
a few friends did visit me, but they still had to keep
their distance. After extended treatments and the
resulting improvement in my health, I was able to
resume the little things in life that I now realize had
greater significance than I thought before my illness.
I embraced watching my children play sports, lying
on the floor building Lego creations with my son,
and working on school projects with my daughter. It
is with deep gratitude for the support of my family,
friends, doctors, synagogue, and community that I
was able to become a better person after my illnesses
than I was before I got sick.

Jerry Rhine

Energy

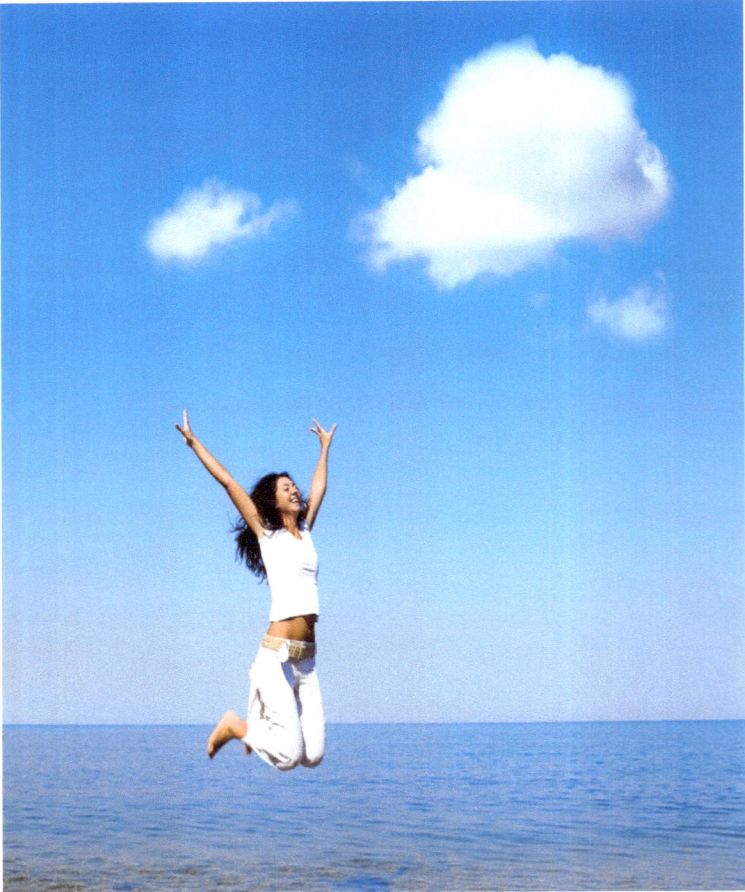

"You can have anything you want if you want it desperately enough. You must want it with an inner exuberance that erupts through the skin and joins the energy that created the world."
— Sheila Graham

Imagine yourself drawing from the energy of the universe. Feel the strength of energy coming down from the sun and up from the center of the earth. Feel a modulated bolt of lightning bring a charge through your body. Feel the flow of a waterfall pull you along.

Practice patience to overcome the fatigue that comes from treatments and chronic disease. Give your body the physical and chemical ability to return your vitality. Allow yourself to bounce back to a comfortable energy level. Draw power from your inner spirit. Take advantage of physical exercise, which is so beneficial to those dealing with cancer and heart disease. Enjoy building stamina while connecting to nature by taking walks. Find a new energetic you.

Ponder that there is positive energy in the universe that we can absorb.

Jerry Rhine

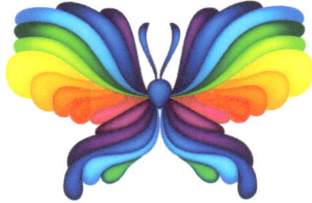

My experience: Due to the side effects of my cancer treatments and the pain medications, I lost a great deal of energy and experienced immense fatigue. It took extraordinary discipline with my visualization practice to regain most of my energy. At times, I would walk to the end of our driveway and be so exhausted that I had to return to the house huffi ng and puffing, ready for a nap. Over time, I began visualizing myself walking all of the holes of the golf course that I played so often. I knew every twist and turn, and could see myself after a great fairway shot or stuck in a bunker. Soon I was able to regain the ability to walk our dogs down the block. I also played 3 holes of golf, then 9 and eventually 18 holes, although I must admit that I now use a cart, partially due to my age.

Spirituality

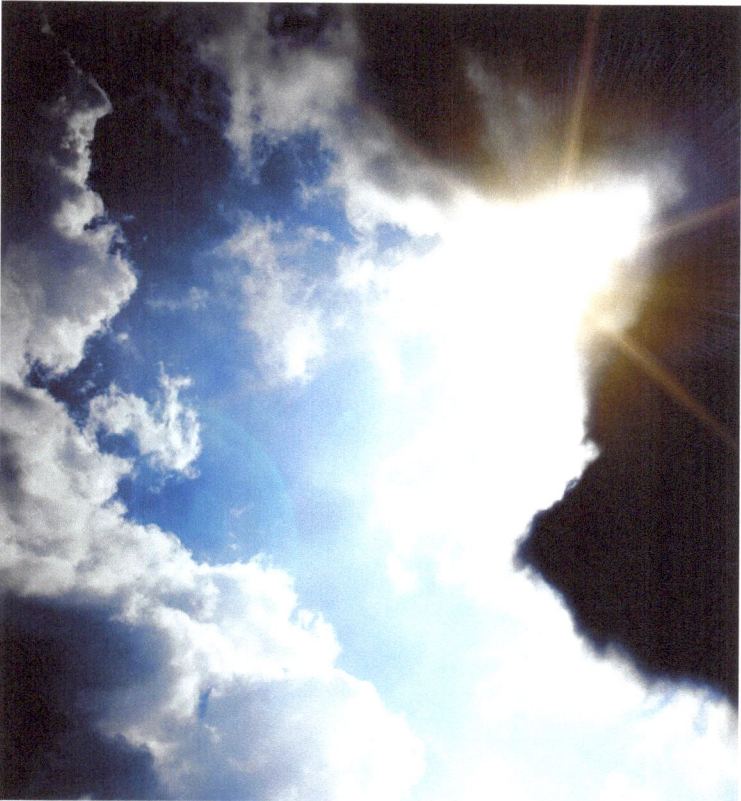

> **"To me, spirituality means 'no matter what.' One stays on the path, one commits to love, one does one's work; one follows one's dream; one shares, tries not to judge, no matter what."**
> *– Yudah Berg*

Affirmation for Spirituality

"I am a loving, kind and forgiving person, in accordance with my spiritual nature."

—Prasanna Vishwasro

Imagine the flame of a candle repeatedly falling, but then rising to the sky. Visualize using your spirit to allow yourself not to be kept down. Imagine your spirit is indomitable. You will not let it be extinguished, and it will remain for all time to be used by those who follow you.

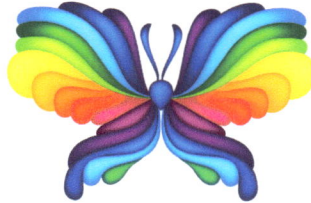

My experience: The spiritual side of me has recovered over and over again after being pushed down by heart attacks, strokes, and cancer. I will not allow my spirit to be snuffed out.

Jerry Rhine

Forgiveness

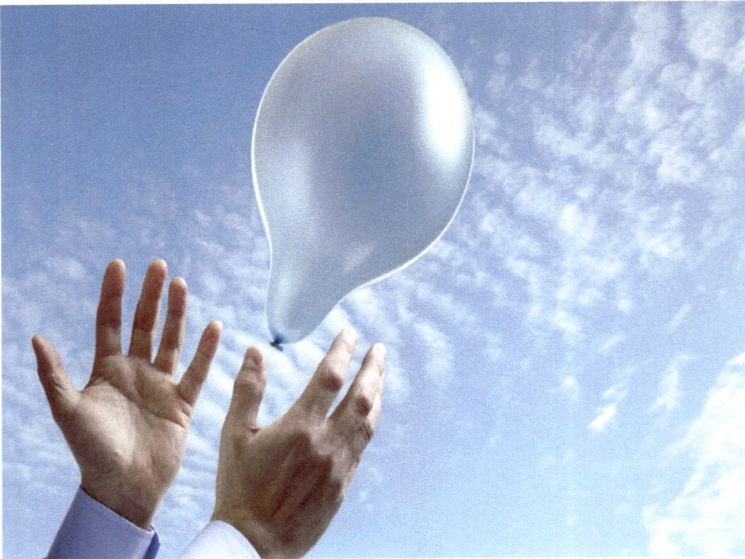

> ## "Forgiveness is the economy of the heart... forgiveness saves expense of anger, the cost of hatred, the waste of spirits."
> *—Hannah More*

Imagine forgiving someone who has hurt you. Feel the grace that comes with forgiveness. Fill a balloon with toxic people who have hurt you. Fill it up further with the destructive feelings of anger and resentment that you have held inside for years. Release that balloon into the sky.

Gain an understanding of those who have caused you trauma and hurt your mind, body, and spirit. This is not an acceptance of damaging acts. Stay aware that you must avoid being with toxic individuals in the future, unless they truly change for the better.

You can heal yourself from abusers of the past by creating a movie. First, visualize a traumatic time and see the facial expressions, dress, location, time of day, and season. Recall what was said and done. Feel all the same emotions.

Now gain understanding of your attacker as a youth. See what love, support, and safety he or she was not given. Imagine yourself teaching this person critical lessons he or she was not taught. Imagine giving him or her love that no one gave that person. Now walk through life with this person.

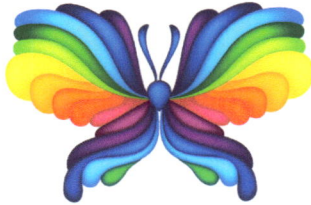

My experience: For years, I carried around a great deal of resentment over the way I was raised and treated by my father. My father was abandoned at age twelve. He lacked the ability to trust people and the world, the ability to handle anxiety, and the ability to understand or give love. He was a verbally abusive alcoholic who controlled his family with an iron hand. After extensive therapy and reflection, I realized that in order to move forward with my physical and emotional health, and be a good father to my children, I had to forgive my father to achieve closure. Learning about spirituality and visualization in Jerusalem enabled me to do that.

Faith

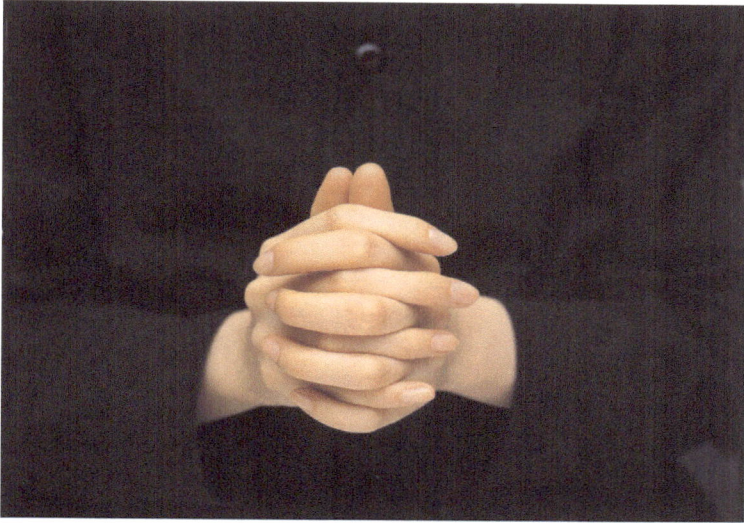

"Faith is a passionate intuition."
— William Wordsworth

Imagine yourself connecting with a Higher Power. Using your imagination, meditate and believe in a good resolution to your situation. Let the light overpower the darkness. In your place of worship, see the stained glass windows and the altar, feel sacramental objects, taste sacramental foods, hear the chanting of psalms and prayers, and be aware of your body as you bow.

Expectant trust, the belief in good outcomes, creates the chemical dopamine. Now faith is being sure of what we hope for and certain of what we do not see. Getting close to God also means loving and using your power to help others and improve the world. Use these experiences in your visualizations. You recall strong emotional ties and memories with the limbic system to create a positive effect. Studies have shown that people who attend religious services heal their cancer better than those who do not attend religious services.

Ponder that our expectations of trust change us physically.

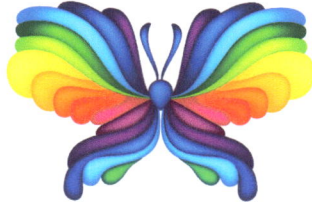

My experience: When I had my first massive heart attack, I experienced a white light. In my unconscious state, I prayed to God that I would live to be there to help my nine month old son and unborn daughter while they grew up. It was a given that I would serve God if I survived. My strong belief in God and positive attitude were essential for my personal healing. I was wandering in a desert of shock and despair having learned that I had lymphoma. I found Chabad of Greenwich. The Chabad organizations throughout the world help those in need of a spiritual connection to God and the community. At this synagogue for learning, I was surrounded by peace and comfort. Praying there has greatly sustained and renewed my faith. The Rabbi at Chabad and the congregants, who are now part of my extended family, were instrumental in my survival.

Jerry Rhine

Giving

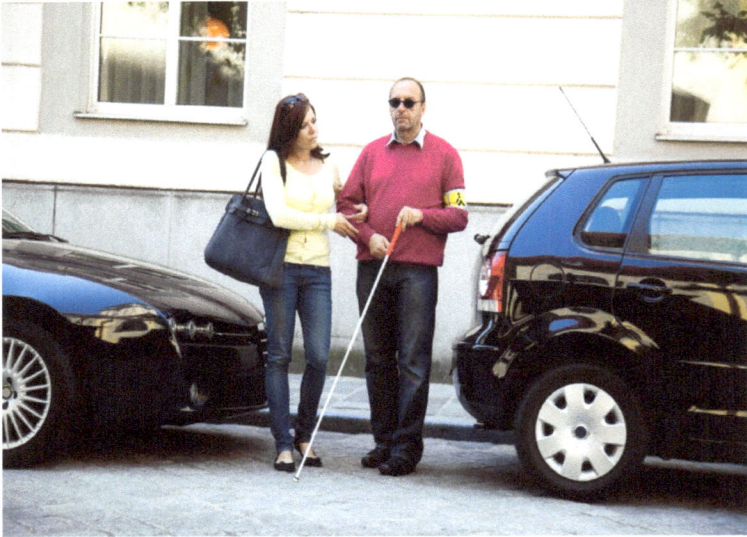

"I don't think you ever stop giving. I really don't. I think it's an on-going process. And it's not just about being able to write a check. It's being able to touch somebody's life."
—*Oprah Winfrey*

Imagine giving to someone in need. Find others who are suffering because of illness, disabilities, economic misfortune, discrimination, or abuse. Have the will to give to others even though you are ill. Call someone else in need so you can both send and receive emotional support.

Ponder that, while only taking from others causes guilt, giving can cause peace, grace, and joy.

Jerry Rhine

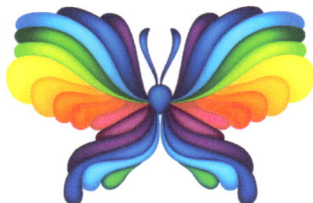

My experience: After chemotherapy and radiation treatments, I realized I wanted to volunteer at Greenwich Hospital since the staff and volunteers were a meaningful part of my recovery. I worked as a volunteer throughout the hospital and amassed over 200 hours trying to help patients regain a positive attitude by accompanying them to treatments, saying a brief hello to someone who seemed down, chatting with someone in a wheelchair, and helping someone who was disabled. This work continues to remind me how far I have come, and how grateful I am to be the person pushing the hospital bed rather than being in it.

Tranquility

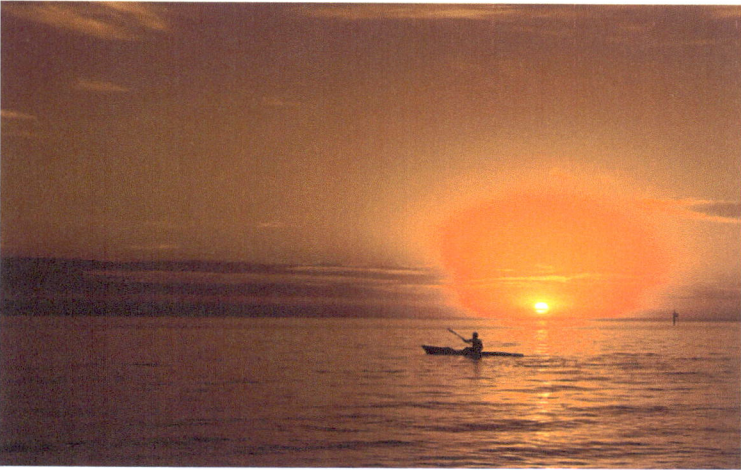

Jerry Rhine

> "The more tranquil a man becomes, the greater is his success, his influence, his power for good. Calmness of mind is one of the beautiful jewels of wisdom."
> – *James Allen*

Imagine yourself in a tranquil situation. Feel the emotional and physical serenity you experience when seeing nature, such as lakes, mountains, the stars in the sky, beaches, and streams. Find yourself in a comforting world, free of anxiety.

Ponder that finding tranquility can lower your blood pressure and relax your muscles and skin. It can increase oxytocin, the hormone for neuromodulation that enables bonding for women, improving attitude and health.

Steve Jobs sought enlightenment and tranquility by studying Zen philosophy. This pursuit included visualizing of nature and doing calligraphy, both of which affected his body, thoughts, and consciousness. Emptying one's mind of clutter makes way for creativity and improves aesthetic experience. In fi nding tranquility, Steve Jobs was empowered to improve the world for humankind.

Savor the moments in the fall when we are surrounded by brilliant colors, hear the rustle of the leaves, and smell the cool autumn air. Savoring is dependent on the keenness of our senses. All of life can be savored rather than experienced mechanically. Meditating is a life-savoring practice that involves a quiet mind.

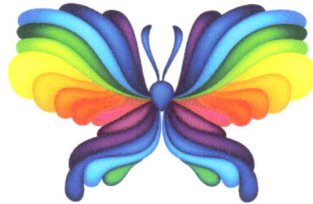

My experience: I enjoy walking on nature trails with friends, while taking in all of nature. I go to the beach. I find tranquility looking at the clouds during the day and the starts at night.

Jerry Rhine

Connection

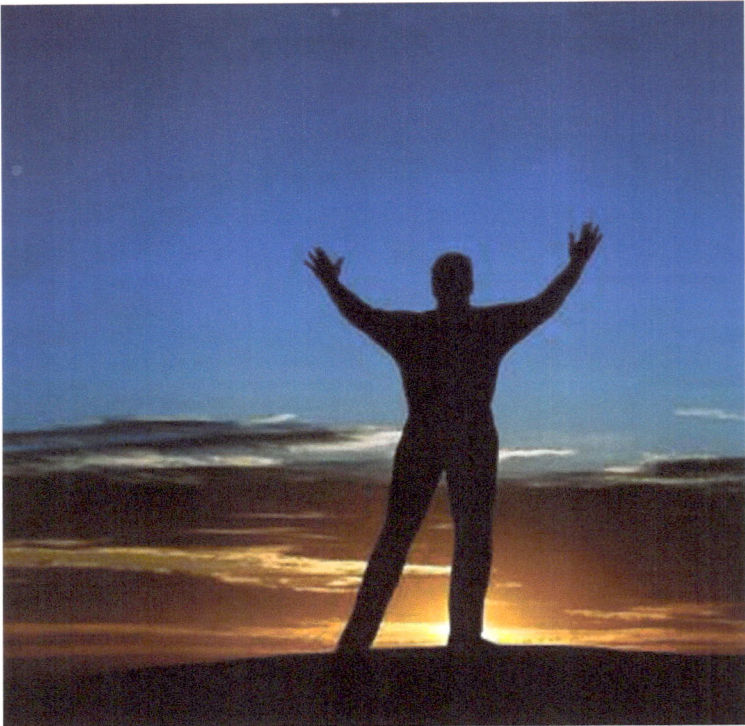

"I'm very close with my higher power. I have a very strong connection with it."
—Fergie

Imagine the feeling of being uplifted by receiving compassion, kindness, care, and forgiveness from your fellowman. Find goodness and love in everyone as you love yourself.

Ponder that studies have shown that people with faith heal better. Visualize connection with God or your Higher Power or positive energy, see a light from heaven filled with love and strength. Surround your body with that light for protection. Allow the light to enter the top of your head and fill all the organs and cells of your body. Let the heat of the light heal the tumors. Feel the cleansing energy of the light both physically and spiritually.

Jerry Rhine

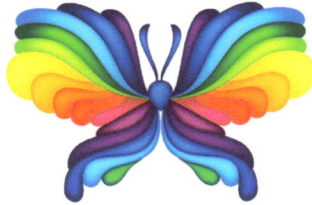

My experience: After I heard I had suffered a heart attack, I fell back into a state of unconsciousness. I asked God to let me survive until my children grew up so I could guide them. Service has become a major part of my life since then.

At age sixty-four, I went to New York University to obtain my Master's Degree in Social Work in order to counsel people with heart disease and work as a spiritual healer to help others. As part of the academic program, I interned at Jacobi Medical Center, which is a public institution in the Bronx, New York, with an eighty percent Hispanic population. While at Jacobi Medical Center, I met and counseled a Catholic Latina woman. She shared with me what she had not shared with other therapists: she was a victim of domestic abuse, and her codependent male partner had left her for a younger woman and taken all the money she had saved from her work. Most importantly, she told me that she intended to commit suicide that evening by taking an Jerry Rhineoverdose of medication. We read psalms, prayed, and cried together. Over time, she healed and found her path working in a day care unit with children. The head of the medical center credited me with saving the woman's life.

Jerry Rhine

Psycho

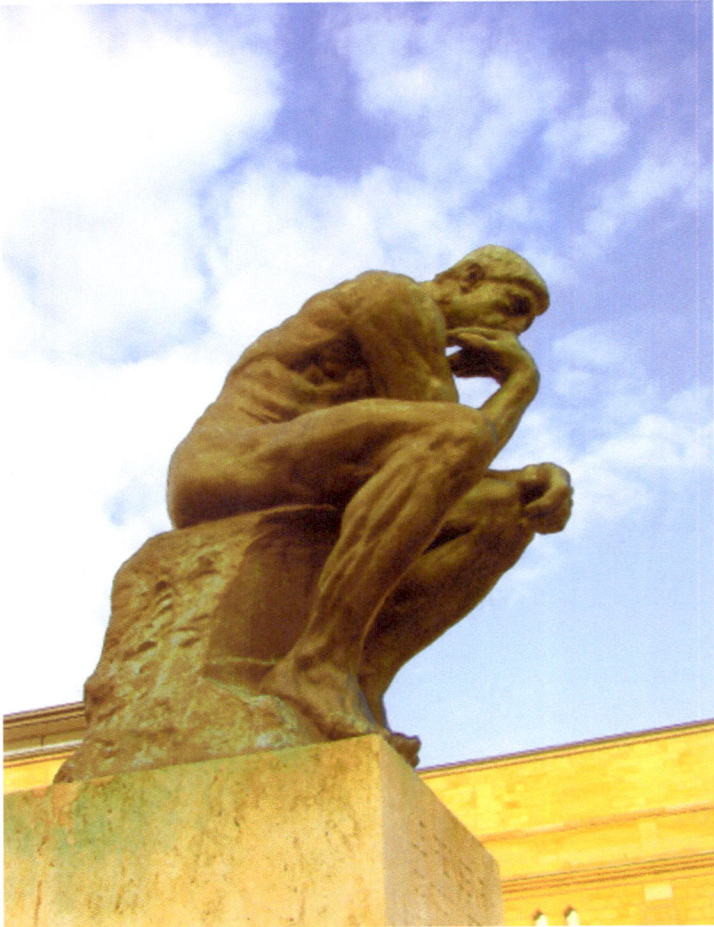

Change, thoughts, feelings, and mood

Neuro

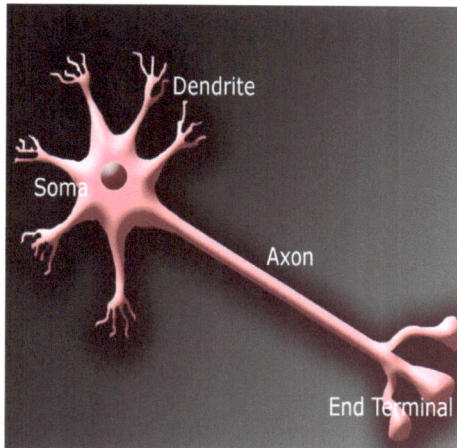

Neurons send signals to other cells by transmitting electro-chemical called, neurotransmitters.

Jerry Rhine

Immunology

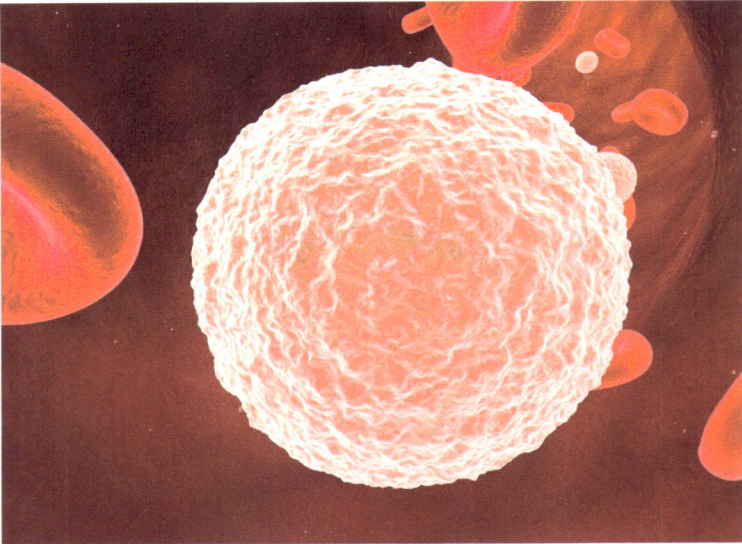

The **immune system** protects against disease by identifying and killing pathogens and tumor cells. Disorders in the immune system, along with causal factors, can play a role in the incidence, metastases, and reoccurrence of cancer.

The Science of Psychoneuroimmunology

The brain and the body are constantly transmitting information in the form of our emotions, which influence the effectiveness of our immune system. Our brain is made of ten trillion transmitters, about as many as there are stars in the galaxy.

These cells are neurons, which transmit negative electrical impulses. Neurons receive information from other cells' processes and send the information to systems in the body, including the immune system. The dendrites of the receptors on the surface of the neuron gather the information in the form of electrical impulses. A combination of this information is sent to the cell body, called the soma and then to axons through nerve impulses. At the end of the axon, chemicals called neurotransmitters are sent across separations called synapses. The neurotransmitters are attached to receptors of specific neighboring dendrites, like a key to a lock. The chemicals such as endorphins, norepinephrine, and dopamine are excitatory; encephalin and GABA are inhibitory. The information received by the receptors will determine the form of the nerve impulse and the firing rate of the next neuron.

A similar process is taking place when hormones are released from our pituitary system.

First, emotional information is gathered in the amygdala, which stores our memories of events. Additional information from our emotions is stored in our limbic system.

How can we affect our mood and enhance our immune system through imagery?

Images are constantly entering our minds both consciously and unconsciously in daydreams and dreams when we sleep. We can alter negative images using pleasant images of our past. These images can be enhanced by bringing in all of our senses. They stimulate emotions encoded in the memory system in our cells. The emotions create electrical impulses and chemicals that travel through our body, communicating interactively with our brain. This communication either suppresses or enhances our immune system.

Imagery of positive and calming emotions can change our negative moods. Positive images enable us to produce better results from medical treatment and curtail the growth and metastasis of cancer cells. They have the potential to reverse heart disease.

Unfortunately, life has dealt you a very difficult challenge.

Biological Factors: Stress

The **immune system, the endocrine system, and the nervous system** are biological systems that prevent and treat cancer. Each is in some manner affected by psychological stress. Even though normal stress alone has not been found to cause cancer, chronic stress that lasts a long time negatively affects a person's overall health and ability to cope with cancer. People who are better able to cope with stress by practicing visualization, have a better quality of life in general. Supplementing visualization with traditional medical treatment for cancer can enhance the chance for recovery.

The **immune system** is a biological system that protects against disease. It detects a wide variety of external agents and distinguishes them from the organism's own healthy tissue, acting as a physical and chemical barrier to infectious agents. Done through a process known as antigen presentation, it identifies and removes foreign substances present in organs, tissues, blood, and lymph nodes utilizing specialized white blood cells.

Among them T cells can recognize and destroy cells displaying tumor antigens and are associated with survival of patients with different cancers.

Disorders of the immune system can result in cancer and heart disease.

The **endocrine system** is the system of glands, each of which secretes different types of hormones directly into the bloodstream to maintain homeostasis. Hormones are substances (chemical mediators) released from endocrine tissue into the bloodstream where they travel to target tissue and generate a response. Hormones regulate various human functions, including metabolism, growth and development, tissue function, sleep, and mood. Tamoxifen is a medication used in hormone therapy to treat breast cancer by blocking the effects of estrogen on cancer cells in breast cancer tissue. Hormone therapy is also used in prostate cancer treatment. Stress can lead to increased levels of hormones such as cortisol, which depresses the immune system. Norepinephrine and serotonin reduce stress levels.

The **nervous system** is integrated with the **endocrine system.** It receives sensory information from its external environment and inputs it to its internal environment. The internal environment integrates this information and transmits signals **to** the central nervous system (CNS) and the peripheral nervous system (PNS). The CNS contains the brain and spinal cord.

The PNS contains a complex network of neurons, nerve cells, which signal to other neurons in the form of electrochemical waves. These signals travel along axons, which are thin fibers. The result is chemicals called neurotransmitters released at junctions called synapses.

These neurotransmitters may be excitatory or inhibitory. Neurotransmitters such as dopamine, acetylcholine, glutamate, and GABA in areas of the brain are involved in the regulation of stress responses. The nervous system enables the body to perceive its external environment and to adapt its performance. At the cellular level, the nervous system is defined by the presence of a special type of cell, called the neuron, also known as a "nerve cell." Neurons have special structures that allow them to send signals rapidly and precisely to other cells.

A cell that receives a synaptic signal from a neuron may be excited, inhibited, or otherwise modulated. The connections between neurons form neural circuits generating an organism's perception of the world and determining its behavior.

Scientists have also found a direct link between our immune system and heart disease. Chronic anxiety or depression suppresses the immune system, producing a higher risk for heart disease and cancer. If we lower our stress levels with our brains, we decrease our risk for heart disease and cancer.

Instructions for Meditation

Go to a quiet place where you will not be disturbed since it is your time to relax. Sit comfortably without crossing your arms and legs. Close your eyes and breathe in and out slowly. Become increasingly aware of your breathing. As you breathe out say the word "one," "om," "shalom," "love," "peace," or a mantra of your choosing. Breathe easily and naturally. Continue for 10 minutes. With practice you will be able to extend the period of this form of relaxation. When distracting thoughts occur, try to ignore them by not focusing on them, and return to repeating your mantra. You are now free from all responsibilities and have nothing to do but allow waves of relaxation to wash through your body. Try and see a light filled with love and power coming down from above from a higher power.

Allow these rays to come into the crown of your head and start to fill up your body. Visualize the light filling every organ, bone, and cell in your body. Let waves of relaxation permeate your entire body and soul.

Now relax the muscles in your forehead and, if necessary, tense your forehead fi rst and then relax it.

Now relax the muscles around your eyes, tensing first if it is helpful. Allow your eyelids to feel very heavy.

Next, allow your mouth to open and your tongue to float in your mouth.

Now relax your nose slowly, breathing in and out.

Swivel your neck slowly, and allow it to relax and rest down to your chest. Shake your shoulders and allow them to relax.

Begin taking deeper and deeper breaths into your chest, exhaling slowly. Imagine breathing into your nose a very comforting steam with a pleasant fragrance.

Breathe the comforting steam into your body slowly and easily. Allow the breathing to happen by itself.

Feel the waves of relaxation moving down your arms. Clench your fi ngers and allow them to relax.

Now let the waves of relaxation travel down the back of your head and along your spine. Let your entire spine bend forward and feel relaxed.

As the sensation of relaxation flows further down your body, allow your buttocks to sink into your chair. Now allow the tension in your legs to disappear.

Shake and relax your ankles. Curl your toes, and allow them to relax.

Shake your entire body looking for areas of tension. Squeeze and relax your muscles. You can imagine that you are a rag doll.

Next feel that your feet are dead weight and your shoes are made of lead.

Imagine a very tranquil and peaceful scene. It can be a lake, or a mountain stream. Bring in all the details of the scene using all of your senses. Perhaps you are by an ocean. Hear the rhythmic pounding of the waves against the sand and rocks, smell the ocean air, see a seagull flying overhead, feel the texture of the sand in between your toes and under your body, and taste the salty spray of the ocean water on your lips. Your mind is at rest. Connect with a higher power or energy.

Suggested Materials

Man's Search for Meaning, by Viktor E. Frankl

Peace, Love and Healing, by Bernie S. Siegel, PhD

Mindful Loving, by Henry Grayson, PhD

Healing Words, by Larry Dossey, MD

Climbing Jacob's Ladder, by Gerald Epstein, MD

Imagery in Healing, by Jeanie Achterberg

Healing of Soul, Healing of Body, by Rabbi Simkha Y. Weintraub

Your Best Life Now, by Joel Osteen

The Relaxation Reponse, by Herbert Benson, MD

National organizations that provide support groups or information.

The American Cancer Society

The American Heart Association

Gilda's Club

Mended Hearts

American Chronic Pain Association

About the Author

Jerry Rhine grew up on Long Island and currently resides in Greenwich, Connecticut. He has been blessed with a loving, compassionate, and supportive family that stood by his side throughout all of his health problems. Jerry's wife is a trusts and estates attorney and a managing partner at Ivey, Barnum, and O'Mara, LLC in Greenwich, Connecticut. She dedicates her free time to serving on the board of direc-tors of various not-for-profit organizations. She also devotes herself to nurturing, supporting, and assisting their children to cope with Jerry's various health problems, which commenced when their eldest child was less than one year old. Jerry's daughter is an art history major at Tufts University who has developed a strong sense of compassion for others by grow-ing up with a chronically ill father. Jerry's son has Tourette Syndrome, and although faced with continual personal chal-lenges has committed himself to volunteerism.

Jerry's son has served as an inspiration. He navigates the world constantly confronted with the ignorance of people who do not understand that tics have no bearing on who he is as a per-son and what he has to offer the world.

Commencing in 1994, Jerry suffered multiple heart attacks and strokes which resulted in severe brain damage, and forced him to discontinue his successful career in commercial real estate. Jerry continues to struggle with organization, memory, and other cognitive functions as a result of the damage to the frontal lobe of his brain.

After a year of cognitive treatment at Burke Rehabilitation Hospital in White Plains, and against the warnings of his therapist that he would fail and become severely depressed, Jerry enrolled at New York University and in 2004 earned a master's degree in social work. During this period, Jerry was diagnosed with prostate cancer and had to undergo various treatments.

After Jerry's graduation from NYU, he was diagnosed with B-cell non-Hodgkin's lymphoma, and is currently in stage three of the disease. He has undergone repeated hospitalizations, surgeries, radiation, including seeding, chemotherapy, cognitive therapy, and physical rehabilitation.

In addition, Jerry was required to use addictive narcotics for extended periods of time in order to cope with the acute pain from his cancers and the resulting treatments. Jerry has been in remission for ten years.

After studying in Israel, Boston, and New York City, Jerry received a certification as a Jewish healer. He is also certified as a Recovery Support Specialist so that he can better provide Peer Support for people who are experiencing the challenges he has met. He has not only survived advanced heart disease and multiple cancers, but Jerry has thrived while helping people from many different faiths to refocus their lives after major health issues and thereby embrace their treatment options in a positive manner with their personal lives.

Jerry has spoken to numerous religious and civic groups, including the American Red Cross regarding coping with life changing illnesses, and has provided his audiences with strategies to empower them and their families to move forward in a productive, constructive, and positive manner. Over the years, Jerry has met with, and been helped by leaders in the area of alternative medicine including Bernie Siegel, who works in the field of cancer, and Dean Ornish, who works in the field of heart disease. Jerry considers himself happy, fulfilled and blessed and intends to continue to move and defy all of the odds.

www.ingramcontent.com/pod-product-compliance
Lightning Source LLC
Chambersburg PA
CBHW041303290326
41931CB00032B/1